JAW SURGERY NUTRITIONAL GUIDE

Complete Guide Unlocking The Secrets Of
Nutrition To Rapid Healing After Surgery
Success, Nourishing Meal Plans, Recipes, Tips
For Optimal Health Wellness)

DR. ALLAN FREDA

Contents

1. Advice from Experts: This book, which was written by nutrition and oral surgery experts with a lot of experience, gives solid advice on what to eat to recover quickly and fully from jaw surgery.

2. Understanding Nutritional Needs: This book talks about the specific nutritional needs of people who have had jaw surgery. It also talks about how important nutrients like protein, vitamins, and minerals are for healing.

3. Recipes for Healing: "Nourish & Heal" has a list of recipes for healing that can help with the healing process. These meals are not only healthy but also tasty, which makes it easier for people to follow their diet plans after surgery.

4. Customised Meal Plans: Customised meal plans make sure that people get the nutrients they need at every stage of their healing by taking the guesswork out of cooking meals.

5. Long-Term Wellness Strategies: The book goes beyond the first few weeks after surgery and gives advice on how to keep your oral health and general health in good shape for a long time.

"Nourish & Heal" is an essential guide that encourages people to take charge of their recovery through proper nutrition and holistic wellness practices, whether they have just been told they need jaw surgery or have already had it done. With its wealth of facts and useful tips, this book is a reliable travel partner on the path to recovery and long-term health.

Disclaimer

The information in this book is for informational purposes only and should not replace professional medical advice, diagnosis, or treatment. Always consult your physician or a qualified health provider regarding any medical concerns. Do not disregard professional medical advice or delay seeking it based on information in this book.

The author does not endorse or have affiliations with any mentioned entities. References are for informational purposes only.

Consult your healthcare provider before making dietary or lifestyle changes, especially during recovery from surgery, as individual needs vary.

Results may vary, and the information provided is not guaranteed to produce specific outcomes.

By reading this book, you acknowledge and agree to consult your healthcare provider before implementing any information herein.

For further guidance, consult your healthcare provider or reputable medical websites for reliable information on surgery recovery diets.

CHAPTER 1

WHAT YOU NEED TO KNOW ABOUT JAW SURGERY AND FOOD

A Look at Jaw Surgery and How It Affects Nutrition:

Orthognathic surgery, which is another name for jaw surgery, is a major treatment that fixes problems with the jaw structure that make it hard to eat, speak, or breathe. During this surgery, the upper jaw (maxilla), lower jaw (mandible), or both are moved around to improve balance and function. The main goal of jaw surgery is to improve the health and function of the mouth, but it also has a big effect on how well a person eats.

The complicated link between jaw structure and nutrition makes it even more important to know how this treatment will affect your nutrition.

One of the main effects of jaw surgery on eating is that it can make it temporarily harder to chew and swallow. Because the surgery includes moving or realigning the jaws, patients may have trouble chewing solid foods or swallowing at first while they are still healing.

This can make it hard to eat a balanced meal and get all the nutrients you need. Additionally, pain and stiffness after surgery can make these problems even worse, so patients need to change what they eat to make sure they get enough nutrition while they heal.

Also, jaw surgery may change a person's general nutritional status because they may change the foods they like and the way they eat. Some people may have changes in how they taste or dislike certain foods after surgery, which can affect the foods they eat and the nutrients they take in.

Also, dietary restrictions or suggestions made by medical workers as part of a patient's post-surgery care plan may affect the kinds of foods they eat, which could affect their nutritional status.

There are effects on a person's nutrition that last longer than the time they are recovering from jaw surgery. These effects may change their eating habits and nutritional state in the future.

For example, people who are getting orthognathic surgery might need to change the way they eat and the foods they eat to account for any long-term changes in how their jaws work or are built. Maintaining optimal nutrition is also important for helping the body heal and avoiding complications after surgery. This shows how important it is for people having jaw surgery to get ongoing nutritional support and advice.

What You Need to Eat Before and After Jaw Surgery:

The nutritional needs of people who are having jaw surgery are very important for making sure that the surgery goes well and that they heal quickly. Making sure you get enough of the essential nutrients you need is very important before and after surgery to help the body heal, avoid problems, and improve your general health.

To make personalized dietary suggestions and help patients achieve optimal nutrition throughout their treatment, healthcare workers need to know about the unique nutritional needs that come with jaw surgery.

Before having surgery on the jaw, patients may benefit from a nutritional assessment and counseling session to make up for any nutrient deficiencies and improve their overall nutritional state in preparation for surgery. Getting enough protein, vitamins, and minerals is especially important right now to help tissues heal, boost the immune system, and improve general health.

In some cases, doctors may suggest dietary supplements or other nutritional treatments to meet specific nutritional needs and make sure that patients get the best nutrition before surgery.

After having surgery on their jaw, people often have to pay close attention to what they eat because their eating habits and nutritional needs change.

 In the early stages of recovery, people may be told to stick to a soft or liquid diet to keep their jaws from getting sore and speed up the healing process. Focusing on easy-to-chew-and-swallow, nutrient-dense foods like pureed vegetables, soups, smoothies, and protein shakes can help make sure you get enough nutrients while still following your postoperative diet limits.

As the healing process goes on and mouth function gets better, patients can slowly switch to a more varied diet with a wider range of tastes and textures. But it's still important to keep eating foods that are high in nutrients and help with healing and general health. Eating foods that are high in protein, vitamins, and minerals, like lean meats, poultry, fish, fruits, veggies, whole grains, and dairy products, can help your body heal properly after jaw surgery by repairing tissues and reducing inflammation.

Along with what you eat, staying hydrated is also an important part of postoperative eating for people who have had jaw surgery. Making sure you drink enough water is important to keep from getting dehydrated, keep tissues moist, and speed up the healing process. Patients should be told to drink a lot of water throughout the day and not drink too much caffeine or alcoholic drinks, as these can make them dehydrated and slow down their healing.

Overall, getting the right nutrition before and after jaw surgery is very important for making sure the surgery goes well and for making the healing process go more quickly. By addressing each patient's unique nutritional needs and giving them personalised dietary advice, healthcare workers can give them the power to make food choices that will help them heal, reduce complications, and improve their long-term health after jaw surgery.

CHAPTER 2

GETTING READY FOR SURGERY ON THE JAW

Jaw surgery, which is also called orthognathic surgery, is a complicated process that fixes problems with the jaw and face structure that are caused by problems with the bones and teeth. Getting ready for jaw surgery is very important for a good result, whether the goal is to fix problems with bite alignment, fix birth defects, or fix obstructive sleep apnea.

People often forget to plan their diet before surgery, but it is an important part of their recovery and healing. This detailed guide will go into detail about what you should eat and how to plan your meals before jaw surgery. It will also talk about what you should have in your kitchen to help you heal as quickly as possible.

Dietary Guidelines and Meal Planning Before Surgery:

Before having jaw surgery, you should follow certain dietary rules and plan your meals to make sure your body is ready for the procedure and the time it takes to heal. Good nutrition not only speeds up the healing process, but also boosts the immune system, lowers the risk of complications, and promotes general health.

Before you go to surgery, you should first talk to your doctor or a registered dietitian about making a personalized diet plan that fits your needs and medical background. In general, you should try to eat a healthy, well-balanced diet that is full of important nutrients like protein, vitamins, minerals, and antioxidants. Getting enough protein is especially important for treating wounds and repairing tissues, so eat lean sources of protein like chicken, fish, tofu, beans, and dairy.

Additionally, make sure you eat a lot of fruits and veggies to get the vitamins and minerals you need to keep your immune system strong and your tissues healing.

Choose a range of colorful fruits and vegetables to make sure you get a lot of different minerals. Whole grains, like brown rice, quinoa, oats, and whole wheat bread, should also be eaten because they give you energy and fiber, which is good for your stomach and bowel health.

You might want to stay away from foods and drinks that can make inflammation worse or cause stomach pain in the days before surgery.

This includes foods that have been processed a lot, sugary snacks, drinks with caffeine, and booze. Instead, choose hydrating drinks like herbal teas, homemade veggie broth, and water to stay properly hydrated and help the body heal itself naturally.

When making meals before jaw surgery, it's best to make soft or liquid meals that are easy to chew and digest because it may be hard to do so after the surgery.

Stock up on healthy foods like soups, smoothies, pureed veggies, yogurt, cottage cheese, and protein shakes so that you have easy access to them while you're healing. Try putting together meals with different tastes and textures to keep them interesting and tasty.

Also, it's important to stay away from restrictive diets and other harsh ways to lose weight before surgery, because getting enough nutrition is key to healing and recovering properly. Instead, focus on feeding your body healthy foods that are full of nutrients that are good for your health and well-being as a whole.

What to Put in Your Kitchen to Get Better:

Due to temporary dietary restrictions and possible problems with chewing and swallowing, it's important to have a well-stocked kitchen after jaw surgery with healthy foods that are easy to make and eat. Planning and organizing your kitchen ahead of time can help you move smoothly into the recovery phase and speed up your body's healing process.

First, stock up on soft, wet foods that are easy on the jaw and don't hurt it. Among these are things like:

1. Bananas, ripe avocados, and canned fruits (in their juice) are all soft fruits.

2. Potatoes mashed, carrots steamed, pumpkin juice, and spinach cooked all the way through.

3. Greek yogurt, cottage cheese, soft tofu, and canned fish (salmon, tuna) are all good sources of protein.

4. You can make instant oatmeal, soft rice, pasta, couscous, and quinoa with grains and carbs.

5. You can use almond milk, soy milk, or rice milk instead of dairy milk.

6. Broths (chicken, veggie, or beef), homemade smoothies (with yogurt, fruits, and vegetables), and protein shakes are all good sources of nutrients.

Make sure you have all the kitchen tools and utensils you need to quickly make and eat soft or liquid-based meals. This could include a mixer or food processor for pureeing foods, a strainer for getting rid of seeds or pulp from liquids, and insulated cups or straws so you can drink without putting too much strain on your jaw.

Also, think about buying pre-packaged foods or meal delivery services that are specifically designed to meet your dietary needs after surgery. This is especially important if you think it will be hard to prepare meals or if you won't have much help while you're recovering. These choices can help you make healthy meals quickly and easily while reducing the stress and work you have to do in the kitchen.

Don't forget to keep hydration tools like reusable water bottles or hydration packs in your kitchen so that you can make sure you drink enough water throughout the day. Staying properly hydrated is important to avoid problems like dehydration, which can slow down the healing process and make recovery take longer.

Lastly, get your support networks, like family, friends, or carers, to help you stock and organize your kitchen so you can get better. Assign chores like grocery shopping, cooking, and cleaning up the kitchen to other people to make your life easier and make sure you have what you need when you need it.

Finally, getting ready for jaw surgery means carefully thinking about what to eat and how to plan your meals so that you can heal and recover as quickly as possible. You can set yourself up for a successful recovery and long-term health by following personalized pre-surgery dietary advice, stocking your kitchen with healthy foods, and organizing your kitchen for ease of use.

CHAPTER 3
RECIPES FOR WET AND DRY FOODS

Jaw surgery, which is also called orthognathic surgery, is a major procedure that tries to fix problems with the jaw, such as misalignment, deformities, or problems with how it works. After surgery, a good diet is very important for speeding up the healing process and helping with recovery. This complete guide is all about what to eat while recovering from jaw surgery. It focuses on recipes for wet and soft foods that are specifically made to meet the nutritional needs of people who are recovering from these procedures.

Smoothies and shakes to help you recover with lots of nutrients

Smoothies and shakes are great for people who have recently had jaw surgery because they contain important nutrients in a form that is easy to digest. You can easily eat these mixed foods that contain vitamins, minerals, proteins, and healthy fats without having to chew or move your tongue a lot. The nutritional worth of these drinks can be raised by adding different things like fruits, vegetables, yogurt, nut butter, and protein powders.

For the best recovery, try adding foods that are high in calcium, protein, and vitamins C and D.

These are important for bone healing and muscle repair. Additionally, adding ingredients that reduce inflammation, like ginger or turmeric, can help lower swelling and pain after surgery.

Making smoothies and shakes with different amounts of liquid or soft fruits can also make them easier to drink.

For example, adding more liquid for a thinner consistency or adding soft fruits for more texture can help. In general, smoothies and shakes are a flexible and healthy choice for people who are still recovering from jaw surgery.

Soups and broths to feel better and get better

Soups and broths are common comfort foods that can help you stay healthy and hydrated while you heal from jaw surgery. These soups and other liquid dishes are great for people with limited jaw movement because they are easy on the throat and full of good nutrients.

Choose broths and soups that are made from scratch with healthy foods like veggies, lean proteins, and whole grains. Bone broth is famous for having a lot of collagen, which helps connective tissues heal and speeds up the healing process generally.

Adding herbs and spices not only makes the food taste better, but they also help the body fight inflammation and germs, which can help with healing after surgery. When making soups and broths, make sure they are smooth by blending or straining them until they are that way.

This will make them easier to eat and keep you from getting sick. Playing around with different flavor profiles and adding a range of items can help keep meals enjoyable and interesting while you're recovering. In the end, soups and broths are a comfortable and healthy choice for people who want to heal quickly after jaw surgery.

Purees and mashed foods that are easy to eat

For people who have had jaw surgery, purees, and mixed foods are great because they are healthy and don't take much work to eat. Because these foods are soft, they are easy on the jaw and throat, making them great for people who are hurting or having trouble eating.

With a blender or food processor, you can turn cooked fruits, veggies, legumes, and grains into smooth and creamy purees. Adding protein sources like tofu, cottage cheese, or cooked lentils can also help keep muscle strength and speed up the healing process.

Adding garlic, herbs, or citrus as a seasoning or flavoring can make pureed foods taste better without losing any of their nutritional value. If you want a heartier meal, mashed potatoes, sweet potatoes, and squash are great options because they are soft and easy to digest while still providing important starches and vitamins.

Also, adding healthy fats like those found in avocado or olive oil can help your body absorb more nutrients and gain more calories. By putting nutrition-dense ingredients first and focusing on texture and flavor, purees and mashed dishes are a satisfying and healthy choice for people who are still healing from jaw surgery.

CHAPTER 4

MEALS PACKED WITH PROTEIN TO HELP YOU GET BETTER

After having surgery on your jaw, a good diet is very important for healing and getting better.

As one of the necessary nutrients, protein is very important for healing damaged tissues, especially muscles.

Meals that are high in protein are an important part of the diet after surgery because they help tissues grow back, wounds heal, and general recovery goes better.

Focusing on high-protein soft foods and looking into vegetarian and vegan protein choices helps make sure that patients get enough nutrition while also taking into account any dietary preferences or restrictions.

After having surgery on your jaw, you need to eat soft, high-protein foods to help your muscles heal and get stronger.

Soft, protein-rich foods are great for nutrition after surgery because they are easy on the healing mouth. Foods like eggs, yogurt, cottage cheese, and tofu can help you get the protein you need without putting too much stress on your teeth.

For even more muscle repair, eating lean foods that are tender and easy to chew, like chicken or fish, is recommended. Not only do these foods provide important amino acids for tissue repair, they also help keep muscle strength while the body heals.

Protein Options for Healing for Vegetarians and Vegans:

For people who follow a vegetarian or vegan diet, getting enough protein after jaw surgery takes careful thought about plant-based sources.

Luckily, many vegetarian and vegan protein choices can help with recovery and healing. Legumes, like lentils, chickpeas, and beans, are great plant-based protein sources that can be added to soups, stews, or drinks to make them healthier.

Nuts and seeds, like walnuts, chia seeds, and hemp seeds, also contain protein, as well as important vitamins and minerals. Tofu and tempeh, which are both made from soybeans, are flexible protein-rich foods that can be used in a lot of different ways.

As a complete protein grain, quinoa makes a healthy base for meals and can be mixed with veggies to make protein-rich, well-balanced meals. By adding these vegetarian and vegan protein sources to their diet after surgery, patients can make sure they heal properly and stay healthy in the long run while still following their preferred eating habits.

A full guide to the best diet for people who have just had surgery or been diagnosed with a new illness. It includes healing recipes, meal plans, and expert advice for long-term health:

After jaw surgery, you need to eat in a variety of ways to help your body heal and stay healthy in the long run. This book has helpful information on how to make the best diet after surgery.

It has healing recipes, customisable meal plans, and expert advice for people who have just been told they have problems with their teeth.

It's very important to understand how nutrition affects recovery because it has a direct effect on how well you heal and your general health.

Patients can speed up their healing and lower their risk of complications after surgery by eating nutrient-dense foods that help repair tissues, reduce inflammation, and boost immune function.

A well-balanced diet with foods from different food groups also makes sure that you get enough of the nutrients you need for healing and long-term health.

People who are going to have jaw surgery can use the information in this complete guide to make smart food choices that will help them recover faster and stay healthy in the long term.

CHAPTER 5

SNACKS AND TREATS THAT ARE HIGH IN NUTRIENTS

Making sure you eat right after having surgery on your jaw is very important for a quick recovery. Nutrient-dense snacks and treats are very important for making sure that the body gets the nutrients it needs to heal and for keeping you comfortable while you're healing.

This detailed guide goes into great detail about how important nutrient-dense snacks and treats are. It gives you ideas for healthy snacks to keep you going and treats to make you feel better and help you recover more quickly.

Ideas for healthy snacks that will keep you going.

Because they are so good for you, snacks that are high in nutrients are very important during the healing phase after jaw surgery. Not only do healthy snacks give you important vitamins and minerals, but they also give you long-lasting energy to fight tiredness and improve your health as a whole. Adding a range of nutrient-dense foods to your diet can help you heal faster and lower your risk of complications.

For snacks, choose foods that are high in protein, like Greek yogurt, nuts, and lean meats. Protein is important for building muscle and repairing tissues. Also, eat a lot of fruits and veggies to get more fiber, vitamins, and antioxidants, all of which help reduce inflammation and keep your digestive system healthy.

Whole grains, like oats and quinoa, are great sources of complex carbohydrates that give you energy that lasts without making your blood sugar go up and down. Eating healthy fats like those found in avocados, olive oil, and fatty fish can also help your immune system work better and lower inflammation. You can improve your diet after surgery and help your body heal faster by picking snacks that are high in nutrients and have a good mix of protein, carbs, and healthy fats.

A lot of nutrient-dense snacks are important for helping the body heal after jaw surgery, but sweet treats can also help you feel better and keep your spirits up during the recovery time.

It's important to eat these treats within limits and keep a healthy diet, but giving yourself a treat every once in a while, can boost your mood and make you feel better overall. For treats that aren't healthy, choose ones that meet your sweet or comfort needs while also being good for you.

So, dark chocolate is a better choice than sugary candies or desserts because it has anti-inflammatory and antioxidant qualities.

Making oatmeal cookies or banana bread at home with whole grain flour and natural sweeteners can be a soothing treat that doesn't have a lot of added sugars or fats that are bad for you.

Nuts, seeds, and dried fruits are full of nutrients that can be added to treats to make them healthier while also giving them more texture and flavor.

To avoid overindulging, remember to enjoy sweets slowly, savoring each bite and focusing on the pleasure they bring. By eating a healthy diet after surgery that includes some sweet treats in moderation, you can take care of your body and your spirit as you heal.

CHAPTER 6

DEALING WITH NUTRITIONAL PROBLEMS

Nutrition is very important for getting better after jaw surgery because it has a direct effect on healing, energy levels, and general health.

Because of how the surgery is done, patients often have problems that make it hard for them to eat a balanced meal. To get the most out of your healing and ensure long-term health, you need to understand and deal with these nutritional problems.

How to Deal with Jaw Pain While Eating:

After having jaw surgery, one of the hardest things for people is having pain in their jaw when they eat. People may have trouble chewing and swallowing food because their jaws may feel sore, stiff, or uncomfortable after the surgery.

Because of this, a lot of patients may lose their appetite or stop eating certain foods altogether, which can make them malnourished and cause problems during their healing.

If you have jaw pain while eating, you need to find ways to make it less painful while still making sure you get enough nutrition. In the days or weeks after surgery, soft or liquid meals are often suggested to ease the stress on the jaw muscles and speed up the healing process.

Smoothies, soups, yogurt, and veggies that have been pureed can give you nutrients without making you chew a lot. Cutting food into small, easy-to-chew pieces and chewing slowly and gently can also help ease pain during meals.

Some people may need pain management methods to get rid of jaw pain and make eating more comfortable. This could include taking painkillers as recommended, using ice packs, or heat therapy to reduce swelling and help the jaw muscles relax.

After some time, physical therapy exercises that are recommended by a doctor can also help restore jaw function and ease pain.

Also, eating foods like fruits, veggies, whole grains, and omega-3 fatty acids that are high in anti-inflammatory properties can help ease pain and speed up the healing process.

The inflammation in the body, including the jaw, can be reduced by eating these foods. They can also help the body's natural healing processes.

Overall, dealing with jaw pain while eating takes a multifaceted approach that focuses on reducing pain, making sure the person gets enough food, and speeding up the healing process.

Patients can deal with this problem better and speed up their recovery by eating soft or liquid foods, learning gentle eating techniques, managing their pain well, and adding anti-inflammatory foods to their diet.

Overcoming texture aversions and food issues is another common nutritional problem that people have after having jaw surgery.

The surgery might change how the jaw feels or moves, which could make it hard to handle some food tastes or consistency's. Because of this, some people may develop dislikes for certain foods or find it hard to find choices that are both healthy and tasty.

It is important to try a lot of different foods and cooking methods that fit different tastes and dietary needs to get over texture aversions and food problems. Trying foods with different tastes, textures, and temperatures can help you find foods that you can handle and enjoy. This could mean making foods smoother by pureeing or blending them, or it could mean adding softer foods instead of harder foods.

Getting help from a trained dietitian or nutritionist can also be very helpful when making changes to your diet and dealing with food problems.

These healthcare experts can give specific advice based on each person's needs, preferences, and nutritional goals. They can also teach you about nutrition, how to plan meals, and how to change recipes so that you eat a healthy, balanced diet.

Adding nutrient-dense foods to your diet is important for getting all the nutrients you need and helping your body heal. To help your body heal, your immune system work better, and your general health, eat a lot of foods that are high in protein, vitamins, minerals, and antioxidants.

Foods like lean meats, fish, poultry, eggs, dairy, legumes, nuts, seeds, fruits, and vegetables are all great sources of essential nutrients that can be changed to fit different taste and texture preferences.

Also, trying different ways to cook, like heating, boiling, or stewing, can help soften foods and make them simpler to chew and swallow. Adding dips, sauces, or gravies can also improve the taste and wetness of food, making it more appealing and fun to eat. Incorporating herbs, spices, and condiments into the diet can also make it more interesting and prevent boredom and routine.

getting over texture aversions and food problems after jaw surgery takes time, effort, and imagination. Patients can get around these problems and keep a healthy, balanced diet while they are recovering by trying new foods, working with their doctors, and focusing on choices that are high in nutrients. People who have had jaw surgery can improve their healing and long-term health with the right diet and support.

CHAPTER 7

GETTING USED TO SOLID FOODS

Getting used to eating solid foods again after jaw surgery is an important part of getting better. After surgery, people often have pain and restricted mobility in their jaws, which makes it hard for them to eat solid foods at first. Because of this, it is important to slowly add solid foods back into the diet to avoid problems and speed up the healing process.

It is very important to slowly start eating solid foods again after surgery so that the jaw can heal properly and the person can get enough nutrition. At first, patients may be given soft foods that are easy to chew, like soups, mashed veggies, and pureed fruits. These foods are easy on the jaw and don't need to be chewed very much, so they cause less pain and strain.

As the patient's jaw gets more mobile and their healing continues, they can slowly start eating harder foods.

When reintroducing solid foods after jaw surgery, it is very important to follow the advice of a doctor or chef. They can make personalized suggestions based on the person's wants and the complexity of the surgery. Patients should also pay attention to their bodies and not rush the process, since going too fast can cause problems or setbacks in the healing process.

During the changeover period after surgery, recipes for soft-chew foods can be very helpful.

These recipes are made to be simple to chew and swallow, which makes them perfect for people whose jaws don't move very easily. Scrambled eggs, yogurt, mashed potatoes, and cooked grains like rice or quinoa are all examples of soft-chew foods. Patients can make sure they are getting the nutrients they need while minimizing pain by adding these meals to their diet.

Soft-chew food recipes can also be changed to fit different diets or personal tastes. For instance, adding tofu or beans, which are high in protein, to soups or purees can help keep muscle strength and speed up the healing process. In the same way, adding different kinds of fruits and veggies to mashed potatoes can help patients get all the nutrients they need to get better.

Meal plans that are specifically made for the time after surgery can help people eat well. Meal plans like these usually have a good mix of soft-chew foods, liquids, and vitamins to make sure you get enough nutrition and help your body heal.

A dietitian or nutritionist can make a personalized meal plan for a person by looking at their nutritional needs, food tastes, and any food restrictions or allergies they may have.

Along with meal plans, it's important to get advice from experts on how to stay healthy in the long run after jaw surgery. Some of these tips could be about keeping your teeth clean, dealing with pain and swelling, and slowly getting back to regular physical exercise. Patients need to carefully follow these suggestions to speed up the healing process and avoid any problems.

Overall, getting used to solid foods again after jaw surgery takes time, planning, and help from medical experts. Patients can make sure they have a smooth recovery and the best healing by slowly adding solid foods, using soft-chew food recipes, sticking to personalised meal plans, and following expert tips for long-term health.

CHAPTER 8
MAKING BALANCED MEALS

Eating well-balanced meals is an important part of getting better after surgery, especially after jaw surgery, where good nutrition is needed to heal and rebuild tissues. It is very important to make meals that meet nutritional needs and work with any dietary limits. Whether you're healing from orthognathic surgery or corrective jaw surgery, your health needs to know how to make balanced meals.

Making healthy meals work with dietary restrictions

Dietary limits can be very different for each person, especially after having jaw surgery. Not being able to eat solid foods, not being able to chew or bite, or needing soft or liquid diets are all common limits. When planning healthy meals around these limits, it's important to pay attention to nutrient density and make sure that every meal gives you the vitamins, minerals, protein, and other nutrients your body needs to heal.

One way to plan meals around dietary limits is to focus on nutrient-dense foods that are soft or easy to chew.

A balanced diet can be achieved by eating a range of fruits, veggies, lean proteins, and healthy fats, even if the person has trouble with some textures or chewing. For instance, making smoothies or soups from blended fruits and vegetables can give you important nutrients in a form that is easy to digest.

There are also special dietary suggestions that you should follow if your doctor or nutritionist gives them to you. They might tell you to stay away from certain foods or chemicals that could slow down or make any problems you have after surgery worse.

By following these suggestions and planning your meals around the foods you can't have, you can help your body heal and recover faster after jaw surgery.

Adding important nutrients to every meal is a key part of helping your body heal and stay healthy after jaw surgery. Protein, carbohydrates, fats, vitamins, and minerals are all essential nutrients.

Each of these nutrients helps the body heal in its way. When planning meals to help you recover from surgery, it's important to focus on foods that are high in these nutrients to help your body heal, your immune system works well, and your general health.

Protein is very important for healing after surgery because it gives tissues the building blocks they need to fix and grow back. Adding lean protein sources like chicken, fish, tofu, beans, and lentils to your meals can help your muscles get stronger and heal faster. Also, eating foods that are high in protein can help you feel full and satisfied, which may be helpful if your hunger is low after surgery.

Another important food that gives the body the energy it needs to heal and recover is carbs.

Choose complex carbs like whole grains, fruits, and veggies. They give you energy and fiber, as well as vitamins and minerals. These carbs are full of nutrients and can help your body digest food, keep your blood sugar levels steady, and give you energy all day.

It's also important to eat healthy fats after surgery because they help control inflammation, make hormones, and absorb nutrients. To improve your health and speed up the mending process, eat foods that are high in healthy fats, like avocados, nuts, seeds, and olive oil. However, it's important to limit the amount of fat you eat because too much can make you gain weight and may not be healthy for everyone, based on their nutritional needs and goals.

Micronutrients, like vitamins and minerals, are just as important for healing after surgery as macronutrients.

Make sure you eat a lot of different fruits and veggies to get enough vitamins and minerals, like calcium, zinc, vitamin C, and vitamin D, which are important for bone health, immune function, and wound healing.

By adding important nutrients to every meal, you can help your body heal and recover faster after jaw surgery. Prioritizing nutrition can help support long-term health and improve outcomes after surgery. You can do this by blending nutrient-rich foods into smoothies, soups, or purees or adding them to soft, easily chewable meals.

CHAPTER 9

IMPORTANT THINGS TO THINK ABOUT FOR HEALING

How well you eat is very important for healing after jaw surgery. A healthy, well-balanced diet can make a big difference in how quickly and well you recover by helping tissues heal, lowering inflammation, and avoiding problems. But some things need to be thought about to get the best diet after surgery and help the body heal the best. This part goes into more detail about specific rules and suggestions for the diet after surgery, focused on what foods to avoid while you're healing and what vitamins and supplements can help.

What to Stay Away from While You Recover

In the early stages of healing from jaw surgery, it's important to stay away from things that could hurt or slow down the healing process. These include chewy, crunchy, or hard foods that can put pressure on the surgery site and cause problems like infection or stitches coming loose. Also, you should stay away from acidic or spicy foods because they can hurt the soft tissues in your mouth and throat, which can cause pain or swelling. Also, things that need to be chewed or moved around the jaw a lot should be avoided so that the healing jaw and muscles around it don't get too tired.

During the early stages of healing, it's best to eat foods that are soft and easy to digest. Some of these are smoothies, yogurt, mashed potatoes, soups, broths, and pureed veggies. If you've recently had surgery, these foods are easy on the wound, don't require much eating, and give you the nutrients you need to heal. To keep the body's healing process going and avoid becoming dehydrated, it's important to drink lots of fluids, like water, herbal teas, and fruit juices that have been reduced.

As the healing process goes on and the mouth starts to feel better, slowly adding back semi-solid and soft foods can help.

But it's important to be careful and pay attention to your body's signals. If there is any pain or soreness while chewing, it could mean that the jaw is not ready for harder foods yet. Professionals in health care or nutrition can give you personalized advice on how to return to a normal diet based on your progress in healing and your specific food needs.

Vitamins and supplements to help the body heal

A healthy diet is important, but some pills and vitamins can also help the body heal and help you get better after jaw surgery. These vitamins might help lower inflammation, speed up tissue repair, and boost the immune system, all of which improve the healing process as a whole. But it's important to talk to a doctor before taking any new supplements, because each person's needs may be different depending on things like the type of surgery they had, any underlying health conditions, and how their medications interact with each other.

Vitamin C is one of the most important products for recovery after surgery because it is a key part of collagen synthesis, a protein that is needed for wound healing and tissue repair. Getting enough vitamin C can help new connective tissue grow and lower the risk of getting an infection.

Citrus fruits, strawberries, kiwi, bell peppers, and broccoli are all high in vitamin C. In some cases, vitamin C pills may be suggested to make sure the right amount is taken in, especially for people who don't get enough vitamin C from their food or who have higher nutrient needs.

Another important nutrient that can help you heal and reduce swelling after jaw surgery is omega-3 fatty acids. Omega-3s can be found in fatty fish like salmon, mackerel, and sardines, as well as in nuts, seeds, and plant-based oils like walnut oil and flaxseed oil.

Individuals who are unable to obtain sufficient amounts from their food or who need extra help with healing and managing inflammation may benefit from taking omega-3 pills.

Protein is an important nutrient for healing after surgery because it helps repair tissues and build muscles. Getting enough protein can help wounds heal faster, keep muscle loss to a minimum, and speed up recovery overall. Lean meats, chicken, fish, eggs, dairy products, beans, nuts, and seeds are all good sources of protein. Protein supplements or meal replacement shakes may be suggested to make sure that people get enough protein, especially those who are having trouble eating or swallowing solid foods while they are still recovering.

To sum up, improving your nutrition during the recovery time after jaw surgery is very important for speeding up the healing process, lowering the risk of complications, and promoting your long-term health.

People can speed up their recovery and improve their general health and well-being by following specific rules about what foods to avoid while they are recovering and by taking supplements and vitamins that help the body heal. Talking to a doctor or nutritionist can give you personalised advice and support to help you get through the post-surgery diet and heal and recover as quickly as possible.

CHAPTER 10
LONG-TERM NUTRITIONAL HEALTH

Long-term nutritional health is an important part of general health and vitality, especially for people who have had jaw surgery. It includes eating habits that will last, keeping your nutrition balanced after you're better, and making food choices that are good for your whole body. Getting the right nutrition is very important for healing, avoiding problems, and staying healthy in the long run. This complete guide will talk about long-term healthy eating habits, why it's important to keep your nutrition in balance after you recover, and ways to achieve long-term nutritional wellness.

Long-Term Eating Patterns for Better Health:
Developing healthy eating habits that last is important for general health and well-being, especially after jaw surgery.

As part of these habits, you choose foods that are good for you and will help you stay healthy over time. Eating a wide range of nutrient-dense foods from all food groups, like fruits, veggies, whole grains, lean proteins, and healthy fats, is an important part of sustainable eating. This makes sure the body gets the vitamins, minerals, and other nutrients it needs to heal, fix tissues, and keep the immune system working well.

Along with focusing on nutrient-dense foods, mindful eating includes things like chewing food well, eating slowly, and paying attention to your body's signals for when you're hungry or full.

These habits not only help your stomach, but they also make you feel full and stop you from eating too much, which can be especially helpful after jaw surgery while you're healing. Also, sustainable eating habits stress how important it is to pay attention to your body's nutritional needs and make changes as needed based on things like your exercise level, health, and personal preferences.

Limiting the amount of processed and refined foods you eat is another part of sustainable eating.

These foods are high in salt, added sugars, and unhealthy fats. Instead, focus on eating whole, barely processed foods that are high in nutrients and don't have any extraneous additives or preservatives. To do this, you should eat a lot of fresh fruits and veggies, whole grains, lean proteins, and healthy fats. By choosing whole foods over processed ones, you can get the most nutrients and improve your health and wellness in the long run.

Keeping the right balance of nutrients after recovery:

While you are healing from jaw surgery, it is very important to eat right. It is also important to keep your diet balanced after you heal for long-term health. To do this, you need to form long-lasting eating habits that are good for your health and well-being.

Making sure you get enough of important nutrients like vitamins, minerals, protein, and fiber is a key part of keeping your nutrition in balance.

Eat a variety of foods from each food group and make sure you get enough fruits, veggies, whole grains, lean proteins, and healthy fats. Getting the nutritional balance is important.

To make sure you get all the vitamins, minerals, and antioxidants you need, try to eat a rainbow of colored fruits and veggies. To help heal and maintain muscles, also eat foods that are high in lean protein, like chicken, fish, beans, legumes, tofu, and tempeh.

Along with focusing on nutrient-dense foods, it's important to watch your portions and not eat too much, since too many calories can cause weight gain and other health problems. Pay attention to your body's signals for hunger and fullness, and stop eating when you feel pleased, not too full. We call this mindful eating.

This can help you avoid eating too much and improve digestion and nutrient intake.

Staying refreshed by drinking lots of water throughout the day is another important part of keeping your nutrition in check. Staying hydrated is important for your health and well-being because water is a key part of many body processes, such as digestion, transporting nutrients, maintaining body temperature, and getting rid of waste. Make an effort to have eight glasses of water each day.

If you are busy or live in a hot place, drink even more.

Besides drinking water, try herbal drinks, infused water, and coconut water as well. They can all help you stay hydrated. Limit your intake of sugary drinks like energy drinks, soda, and fruit juice because they can make you eat too many calories and not give you much nutrition. Instead, drink water or other low-calorie drinks to stay refreshed and improve your health and well-being as a whole.

Overall, keeping your nutrition in balance after you've recovered means making eating habits that will last and help your health and well-being in the long run. Prioritizing nutrient-dense foods, practicing mindful eating, watching your portion sizes, and drinking plenty of water can help you get the most nutrients and improve your health over time.

CONCLUSION

To fully recover from surgery and stay healthy in the long run, you need to take a multifaceted approach that includes nutrition, lifestyle changes, and professional help. This complete guide is a treasure trove of information. It includes not only healing recipes and meal plans made just for people who have just been diagnosed, but also useful insights and expert tips to help you stay healthy.

We have learned a lot about the ins and outs of a post-surgery diet and how important it is to fuel the body with nutrient-dense foods to speed up recovery and improve general health. People can not only speed up their recovery but also set themselves up for long-term health and energy by adopting a balanced and personalized approach to nutrition.

Additionally, the addition of meal plans and recipes provides useful assistance, making it simpler for people to make dietary changes and follow suggested rules. These resources are meant to give people the tools they need to get healthy by giving them motivation and direction at every step of the way.

But it's important to remember that the best way to recover from surgery isn't just to watch what you eat. Lifestyle choices like getting enough rest, managing stress, and being active all play important parts in helping the body heal and stay healthy over time.

People need to take a complete approach to their health and well-being, which means looking at all of them.

When it comes down to it, getting better after surgery and staying healthy in the long run is an ongoing process that needs commitment, patience, and self-care. People can start on the path to healing, vitality, and a better, healthier future by following the guidelines laid out in this comprehensive guide and using the tools it offers.

www.ingramcontent.com/pod-product-compliance
Lightning Source LLC
Chambersburg PA
CBHW070323290526
45791CB00003B/1238